Table of Contents

Author's Notes - 3

Forward - 4

Introduction - 5
Reusi Dat Ton: The Thai Hermit's Exercises - 5
The Tree of Physical Yogas - 6
Foundations of Traditional Thai Massage - 7
Reusi Dat Ton in Traditional Art - 8
Textual Sources of Reusi Dat Ton - 9
The Benefits of Reusi Dat Ton - 11

Self Massage - 13
Face - 14
Neck - 17
Shoulders - 19
Arms - 21
Hands - 23
Torso & Back - 24
Legs - 27
Feet - 31
Sen Lines of Northern Thai "Lanna" Massage - 33

Joint Mobilization - 34
Seated Joint Mobilization - 35
Lower Body - 36
Torso - 36
Upper Body - 38
Neck & Head - 40
Standing Joint Mobilization - 43
Neck & Head - 44
Upper Body - 45
Torso - 48
Lower Body - 50

References - 52

"Self-Massage and Joint Mobilization of Traditional Thai Yoga: Reusi Dat Ton Part 1 Handbook"
by David Wells

Text and Photos Copyright © 2016 by David Wells except where otherwise noted.

Parts of this book were previously published in the article "Reusi Dat Ton: The Thai Hermit's Exercises" in Yoga Mimamsa, July 2012, Volume XLIV, No.2, Kaivalyadhama, Lonavala, India.

All rights reserved. No part of this book may be reproduced or transmitted in any form or by any means, digital, electronic or mechanical, including photocopying, recording, or by any information storage and retrieval system, without permission in writing from the author.

All Rights Reserved

ISBN-13: 978-1533201010

ISBN-10: 1533201013

LCCN: 2016907948

CreateSpace Independent Publishing Platform, North Charleston, SC

Author's Notes

Thanks to the following people who helped make these Handbooks possible: my *Reusi Dat Ton Models:* Sarah Carl, Laura Covington, Julia Henry, Deborah Hodges, Matthew Holton, Satya Larrea, Jack Maxwell, Randi Morrison, and Erin Wright; to Linley Eathorne, Jill & Grace Harman, and Sherian Thomas for photography and special assistance; to Elaine Esquibel for editing; to Dusnee Mathison for translation; to Oscar de Cárdenas for graphic design; to Sarah Carl, Romina Correa, Jessica Dafni, Oscar de Cárdenas, Enrique Dianti, James Galusha, James Hooker, Laura Iwasetschko, Nephyr Jacobsen, Ulric Legouest, Sunny Nilchavee, Fabian Novellino, Kristin Nuttall, Gregory Oed, Pierce Salguero, Mr. Shirpurkar, Delfina Sommerville, Hemali Thakkar, Dustin Williams, and Jennifer Vanderburg for advice, and to Danko Lara Radic, Caitlin Ryan, Reusi Prasanga Samavajra, and Heath Reed for Charts, Illustrations, and Photos.

Special Thanks to my teachers and their teachers: Dr. Ajahn Prasong Sompetch, *"Grandfather"* in Chiang Mai, Reusi Tevijjo, and the late Ajahn Pisit Benjamongkonware for having the Wisdom to learn, preserve, and pass on the wonderful Tradition of *Reusi Dat Ton* which was nearly lost to our modern world.

Finally an extra special Thanks to my primary teacher, Reusi Tevijjo, for generously sharing with me the mysteries of this rare gem. In truth, these books are as much his as they are mine.

This Handbook "Self Massage and Joint Mobilization of Traditional Thai Yoga: Reusi Dat Ton Part 1" is the first in a series of Handbooks which will cover the full range of practices of "Reusi Dat Ton" or Traditional Thai Yoga. Future volumes will include "Basic Exercises and Breathing of Traditional Thai Yoga: Reusi Dat Ton Part 2" and "The Complete Guide to Traditional Thai Yoga: Reusi Dat Ton Part 3".

The techniques, ideas, and suggestions in this book are not intended as a substitute for proper medical advice. Consult your physician or health care professional before beginning this or any new exercise program, particularly if you are pregnant or nursing, if you are elderly, or if you have any chronic or recurring physical conditions. Any application of the techniques, ideas, and suggestions is at the reader's sole discretion and risk.

— David Wells

Forward

"It brings me much happiness to see these books finally ready to be shared with the world. David has spent many years traveling throughout Asia seeking teachers who would share with him the ancient tradition of Reusi Dat Ton. This information is incredibly difficult to find. What little Reusi Dat Ton information that has previously been accessible to the general public — both in Asia and the West — has been largely superficial and inconsistent. Through much effort and dedication, David has successfully created a thorough guide to the Reusi Dat Ton practices that honors their ancient roots and adheres to the traditional methods through which they have been preserved for hundreds of years.

My teachers have long spoken of the importance of preserving the knowledge of their lineage and of doing so in the most traditional methods possible. As modern society rockets ahead, so many traditional practices have been scattered or lost, disappearing as the last lineage holders pass on. Preserving practices such as Reusi Dat Ton is more important than ever as we near the tipping point where we risk losing these traditions forever. For this reason, I have been very happy to support David on this project and share with him what little knowledge I have from my own Reusi Dat Ton studies and practices.

David's efforts have resulted in a rich resource for this little known and often misunderstood tradition. These books will benefit many who have long sought to learn more about these practices as well as those who are yet to discover them. It is my hope that by sharing this information, David has opened the door for greater understanding and exploration of Reusi Dat Ton and the greater traditions from which it came."

— **Reusi Tevijjo**, Chiang Mai, Thailand

Introduction

Reusi Dat Ton: The Thai Hermit's Exercises

Reusi Dat Ton is a little known aspect of traditional Thai healing and culture. It consists of breathing exercises, self-massage, dynamic exercises, poses, mantras, visualization, and meditation.

"Reusi" in Thai, from the Sanskrit *Rishi*, is an Ascetic Yogi or Hermit. "Dat" means to stretch, adjust, or train. "Ton" is a classifier used for a Reusi and also means oneself. So "Reusi Dat Ton" means the Hermit's or Yogi's self-stretching or self-adjusting exercises. Reusis were also known as "Jatila," "Yogi," and "Chee Prai." The Reusis were custodians and practitioners of various ancient arts and sciences such as: tantra, yoga, natural medicine, alchemy, music, mathematics, astrology, palmistry, etc. They have counterparts in many ancient cultures such as: the Siddhas of India, the Yogis of Nepal and Tibet, the Immortals of China, the Vijjadharas of Burma, and the Cambodian Eysey (from the Pali word for Reusi, *Isii*)

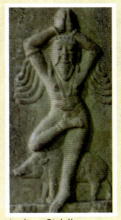
Indian Siddha

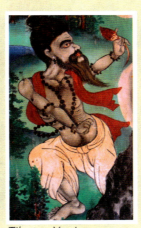
Tibetan Yogi

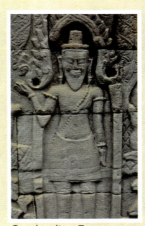
Cambodian Eysey

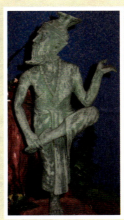
Thai Reusi

There are different Reusi traditions within Thailand. There is a Southern Thai/Malay Tradition, a Northeastern Thai/Lao Tradition, a Central Thai/Khmer Tradition, and a Northern Thai/Burmese/Tibetan Tradition. In Thailand, there are Reusis as far South as Kanchanaburi Province who follow the Northern Thai/Burmese/Tibetan Reusi Tradition.

A typical Reusi Dat Ton program would begin with breathing exercises and self-massage, followed by dynamic exercises and poses (some of which involve self acupressure), and finish with visualization, mantras, and meditation. The exercises and poses of Reusi Dat Ton range from simple stretches that almost anyone could do to very advanced poses which could take many years to master.

Part I: Self-Massage & Joint Mobilization

INTRODUCTION – TREE OF PHYSICAL YOGAS

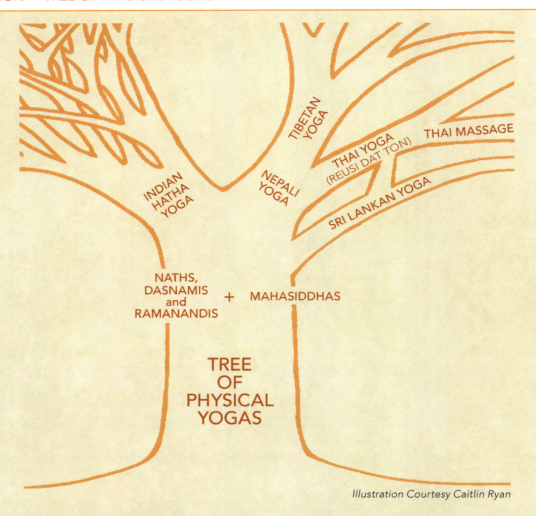

Illustration Courtesy Caitlin Ryan

"Yoga is not a single tradition, but a family of self-cultivation traditions that are widespread across India, Tibet, and Southeast Asia. They typically involve a tantric view of the relationship between body, mind, and spirit being managed through "energies" (usually understood as winds), and they typically involve a combination of meditation, breathing exercises, and physical postures to manage these "energies". With this definition of yoga, then one can simply say that "Reusi Dat Ton" is a Thai form of yoga." – Pierce Salguero PhD.

The Tree of Physical Yogas

Imagine for a moment, a "Tree of Physical Yogas" with its different branches representing the different Yoga traditions that have developed over the centuries. Today the most well known branch is that of Indian Hatha Yoga with its numerous smaller branches representing the many different modern styles which were developed out of the Traditional Medieval India Hatha Yoga of the Nath Yogis, Dasnami Naga Samnyasis and Ramanandi Tyagis. Other lesser-known but equally important branches of the Yoga Tree include Tibetan Yoga and it's various forms such as: Yantra Yoga, Kum Nye, Tsa Lung, Lu Jong, Tumo, etc. There is also the Thai Yoga or "Reusi Dat Ton" Branch and the tradition of Thai Traditional Massage that was developed out of "Reusi Dat Ton." Other cultures also had their own unique systems of Yoga practices, including Nepal and Sri Lanka, whose traditions also influenced the Thai.

Some of the Reusi Dat Ton techniques are similar to, or nearly identical to, some techniques in various Tibetan Yoga Systems particularly, "Yantra Yoga," "Kum Nye", and the Tibetan Yoga Frescoes from the

Lukhang Temple behind the Potala Palace in Lhasa Tibet. (See Norbu, Tulku, and Baker) For example: some of the self massage techniques, exercises, poses, neuromuscular locks (bandhas in Sanskrit), breathing patterns, ratios, visualizations, and the way in which male and female practitioners would practice the same technique differently are almost identical. It is possible that Reusi Dat Ton and some of the Tibetan Yoga Systems are derived from a common source, which Rishis brought with them as they moved down the Himalayan foothills into Southeast Asia.

Foundations of Traditional Thai Massage

According to the Reusi Tevijjo:

> *"The foundation and key to Traditional Thai massage is Reusi Dat Ton. Ancient Reusis, through their own experimentation and experience, developed their understanding of the various bodies (physical, energetic, psychic, etc). They discovered the postures, channels, points, the winds, and wind gates within themselves. Later it was realized that these techniques could be adapted and applied to others for their healing benefit, which is how Thai massage was developed. So, in order to really understand Thai massage, as a practitioner, one should have a foundation in Reusi Dat Ton and be able to experience it within oneself and then apply it to others. It is not only the roots of Thai massage but it also unlocks the method for treating oneself and maintaining one's own health."*

It is also interesting to note that there are many close similarities between certain Thai massage techniques. *Reusi Dat Ton* exercises and some of the Indian Hatha Yoga therapeutic warming up exercises (the *Pawanmuktasana* or wind liberating and energy freeing techniques). There is even an advanced Hatha Yoga pose, *Poorna Matsyendrasana*, which compresses the femoral artery and produces the same effect as "opening the wind gate" in Thai massage. (Saraswati)

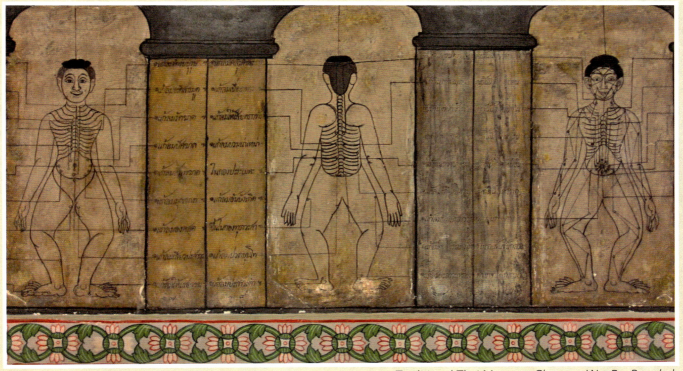

Traditional Thai Massage Charts at Wat Po, Bangkok

Part 1: Self-Massage & Joint Mobilization

Reusi Dat Ton in Traditional Art

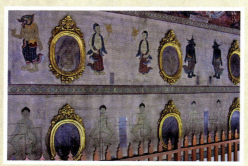

In 1767, invading Burmese armies destroyed the old Thai capital of Ayutthaya. Soon after his coronation in 1782, the Thai King Rama I established a new capital in what is today Bangkok. He initiated a project to revive the Thai culture after the disaster of Ayutthaya. An old temple Wat Potharam, (popularly known as "Wat Po"), was chosen to become the site of a new Royal temple and formally renamed Wat Phra Chetuphon. Beginning in 1789, a renovation and expansion project was begun on the temple. King Rama I also initiated a program to restore and preserve all branches of ancient Thai arts and sciences including: medicine, astrology, religion, and literature. As part of this project, medical texts from across the kingdom were collected and brought to be stored at Wat Po. The King also ordered the creation of a set of clay Reusi statues depicting various Reusi Dat Ton techniques.

Engraved Medical Tablets

This restoration project was continued by the Kings Rama II and Rama III. As part of this work, scholars compiled important texts on various ancient arts and sciences and created authoritative textbooks for each of these fields. In 1832, a project to etch the medical texts into marble tablets was begun. Medical theories regarding the origin and treatment of disease, massage charts, and over 1000 herbal formulas were all recorded on the marble tablets. Gardens of medicinal herbs were also planted on the temple grounds. Thus, Wat Po was to become "a seat of learning for all classes of people in all walks of life" which would "expound all branches of traditional knowledge both religious and secular", and serve as "an open university" of traditional Thai culture with a "library of stone". (Griswold, 319-321)

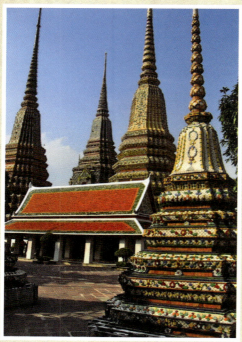

Wat Po

By 1836, the clay Reusi Dat Ton statues created by order of King Rama I had deteriorated. To replace these, King Rama III commissioned the creation of 80 new Reusi Dat Ton statues. Each statue depicted a different Reusi performing a specific Reusi Dat Ton technique. For each statue there was a corresponding marble tablet upon which was etched a poem describing the technique and it's curative effect. These poems were composed by various important personalities of the day. Princes, monks, government officials, physicians, poets, and even the King himself contributed verses. The original plan was to cast the statues with an alloy of zinc and tin, but unfortunately only the more perishable material stucco was used. The statues were then painted and housed in special pavilions. Over the years most of the original statues have been lost or destroyed. Today only about 20 remain and these are displayed upon two small "Hermit's Mountains" near the Southern entrance of Wat Po. The marble tablets have been separated from their corresponding statues and are now stored in the pavilion Sala Rai.

INTRODUCTION – TEXTUAL SOURCES OF REUSI DAT TON 9

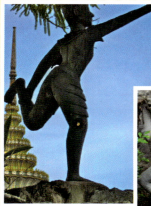
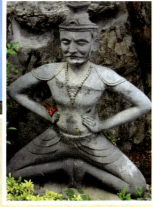

Reusi Dat Ton Statues at Wat Po

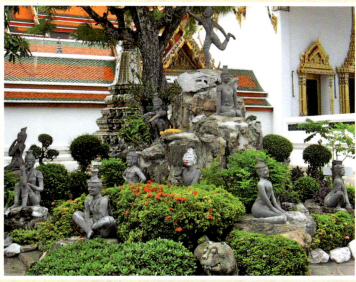

"Hermit's Mountain" Wat Po

Textual Sources of Reusi Dat Ton

We may never know what, if any, ancient texts on Reusi Dat Ton may have existed and were lost when the invading Burmese armies destroyed the old Thai capital of Ayutthaya in 1767. Today, the closest thing to an original source text on Reusi Dat Ton is an 1838 manuscript commissioned by Rama III entitled *The Book of Eighty Rishis Performing Posture Exercises to Cure Various Ailments*. Like other manuscripts of the time, this text was printed on accordion like folded black paper, known in Thai as "Khoi". This text, popularly known as the *Samut Thai Kao* features line drawings of the 80 Wat Po Reusi Dat Ton statues along with their accompanying poems. In the introduction, it states that Reusi Dat Ton is a "...system of posture exercises invented by experts to cure ailments and make them vanish away". (Griswold, 321) This text is housed in the National Library in Bangkok. There are also other editions of this text housed in museums and private collections as well.

The *Samut Thai Kao* follows an old tradition also found in ancient Indian, Nepali, and Tibetan Yoga manuscripts that list 80 to 84 different techniques. The *Samut Thai Kao* is, however, only a partial collection of all the various Reusi Dat Ton techniques. A 1958 Wat Po publication, *The Book of Medicine,* includes a section on Reusi Dat Ton. While it contains verses based upon the poems at Wat Po, many of the accompanying illustrations depict completely different techniques. There are also a few modern day Reusis such as Reusi Prasanga Samavajra who continue the ancient tradition of recopying by hand old Reusi Dat Don manuscripts which have been passed down over the centuries through their lineage.

In the Southern Thai town of Songkhla, on the temple grounds of Wat Machimawat, is a pavilion known as the "Sala Reusi Dat Ton".

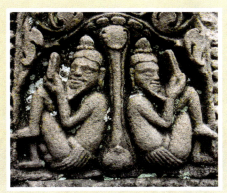

Reusis from Prasat Phnom Rung, Buriram

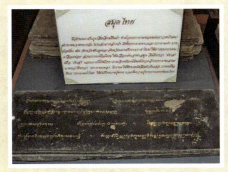

Traditional Thai Manuscript

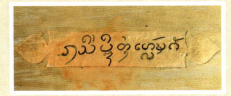

Rare "Reusi Dat Ton" text hand copied by Reusi Prasanga Samavajra

Part I: Self-Massage & Joint Mobilization

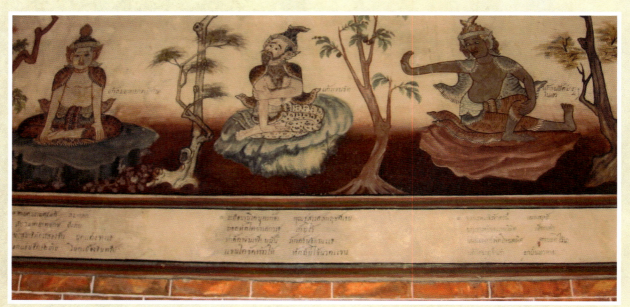

Reusi Dat Ton Mural at Wat Machimawat

High up on the inside walls of this pavilion is a mural which depicts 40 of the Reusi Dat Ton techniques along with the accompanying poems from the *Samut Thai Kao*.

There is a special section devoted to Thai Medical History at the Mahidol University's Siriraj Medical Museum on the Bangkok Noi campus in Bangkok. There, one can view a Reusi Dat Ton display featuring small painted wood Reusi figures that depict over 60 different Reusi Dat Ton techniques. This display is based upon the 1958 Wat Po text *The Book of Medicine*.

In Nonthaburi, on the Ministry of Public Health Campus at the Institute of Thai Traditional Medicine, there is the Thai Traditional Medicine Museum. Inside the museum is a small display of Reusi Dat Ton statues. Outside the museum is an artificial mountain upon which have been placed various Reusi statues demonstrating Reusi Dat Ton techniques. Within the mountain is the "Hermit's Cave" which houses numerous small Reusi statues also depicting Reusi Dat Ton techniques. These statues depict techniques from both the *Samut Thai Kao* and *The Book of Medicine*.

On the outskirts of Bangkok, in the town of Samut Prakan, is the cultural park, the Ancient City or "Muang Boran". One of the many attractions is a "Sala of 80 Yogi" which features 80 life-sized Reusi statues illustrating various Reusi Dat Ton techniques. There are even depictions of Reusi Dat Ton techniques not found in either of the two Wat Po texts.

Students of Reusi Dat Ton should bear in mind that while some of the Reusi Dat Don statues, drawings, paintings, and poems are beautiful works of art, they were created by artists who were not necessarily all practitioners of Reusi Dat Ton. In fact, a number of images do not illustrate the actual techniques entirely accurately. Even in 1836, there was some uncertainty as to which technique produced which effect and some poems were used for more than one technique. Therefore, students of Reusi Dat Ton should also seek out living teachers who have learned from authentic sources such as actual Reusis who can teach the techniques in their authentic form.

There are also additional Reusi Dat Ton techniques practiced by Reusis today, which are not found in any text, nor depicted in any sculpture or paintings. These are also traditional techniques, which have been passed down from teacher to student over the centuries. There are close to 300 different exercises and poses, including variations, in the entire Reusi Dat Ton System.

The Benefits of Reusi Dat Ton

In both the *Samut Thai Kao* and *The Book of Medicine,* the texts not only describe the techniques, but also ascribe a therapeutic benefit to each pose or exercise. Some poems describe specific ailments while others use a mix of Sanskrit, Pali, and Traditional Thai Medical terminology.

Some of the ailments mentioned include: abdominal discomfort and pain, arm discomfort, back pain, bleeding, blurred vision, chest congestion, chest discomfort and pain, chin trouble, chronic disease, chronic muscular discomfort, congestion, convulsions, dizziness and vertigo, dyspepsia, facial paralysis, fainting, foot cramps, pain and numbness, gas pain, generalized weakness, generalized sharp pain, headache and migraine, hand discomfort, cramps and numbness, heel and ankle joint pain, hemorrhoids, hip joint problems, joint pain, knee pain and weakness, lack of alertness, leg discomfort, pain and weakness, lockjaw, low back pain, lumbar pain, muscular cramps and stiffness, nasal bleeding, nausea, neck pain, numbness, pelvic pain, penis and urethra problems, scrotal distention, secretion in throat, shoulder and scapula discomfort and pain, stiff neck, thigh discomfort, throat problems, tongue trouble, uvula spasm, vertigo, waist trouble, wrist trouble, vomiting, and waist discomfort.

Some of the Ayurvedic disorders described in the texts include: Wata (Vata in Sanskrit) in the head causing problems in meditation, severe Wata disease, Wata in the hands and feet, Wata in the head, nose, and shoulder, Wata in the thigh, Wata in the scrotum, Wata in the urethra, Wata causing knee, leg, and chest spasms, Wata causing blurred vision, Sannipat (a very serious and difficult to treat condition due to the simultaneous imbalance of Water, Fire, and Wind Elements which may also involve a toxic fever) an excess of Water Dhatu (mucous), and "Wind" in the stomach. Other benefits

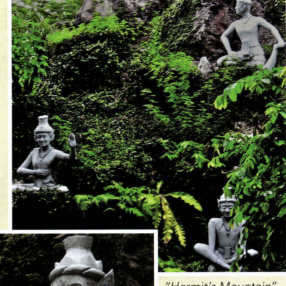

"Hermit's Mountain" at The Thai Ministry of Public Health

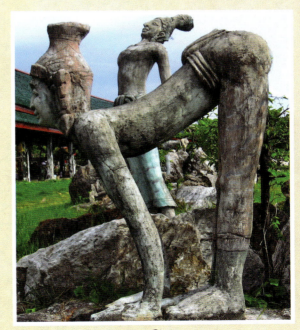

Reusi Statue at Ancient City

Part I: Self-Massage & Joint Mobilization

INTRODUCTION – THE BENEFITS OF REUSI DAT TON

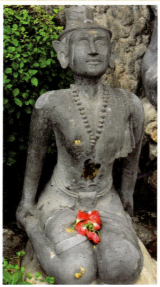
For Shoulder Discomfort

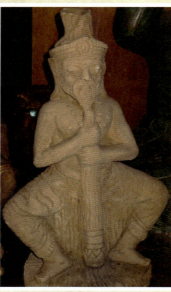
For Foot Cramps & Longevity

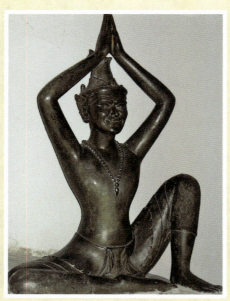
For Headache

described in the old texts include increased longevity and opening all of the "Sen". (Various types of "Sen" or channels are found in Traditional Thai Medicine. There are Gross Earth Physical "Sen" such as Blood Vessels. There are also more Subtle "Sen" such as channels of Bioenergy flow within the Subtle Body, known as "Nadis" in Sanskrit as well as channels of the Mind.)

In recent years, the Thai Ministry of Public Health has published several books on Reusi Dat Ton. According to these modern texts, some of the benefits of Reusi Dat Ton practice include: improved agility and muscle coordination, increased joint mobility, greater range of motion, better circulation, improved respiration, improved digestion, assimilation and elimination, detoxification, stronger immunity, reduced stress and anxiety, greater relaxation, improved concentration and meditation, oxygen therapy to the cells, pain relief, slowing of degenerative disease, and greater longevity. (Subcharoen, 5-7) A recent study at Naresuan University in Phitsanulok, Thailand, found that after one month of regular Reusi Dat Ton practice there was an improvement in anaerobic exercise performance in sedentary females. (Weerapong et al, 205)

What follows are the Self Massage and Joint Mobilization Exercises of Traditional Reusi Dat Ton. My students and I have found these seemingly simple techniques to be profoundly therapeutic and beneficial. These exercises will also prepare one for the more advanced techniques which will be introduced in Parts 2 and 3 of these "Reusi Dat Ton" Handbooks.

Always remember: **DO NOT HURT YOURSELF!** If you find that a technique is uncomfortable or painful, skip it and move on to another technique. Everyone is different and not every technique will be appropriate for everyone.

Traditional Thai Yoga "Reusi Dat Ton"

Self Massage

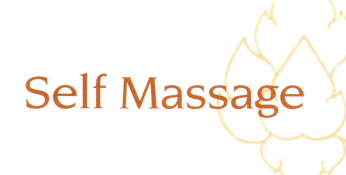

If time is short and one is unable to do the Full Body Self Massage, one could just do the Head & Neck and then massage any specific problem areas. One can also do self-massage between exercises as needed.

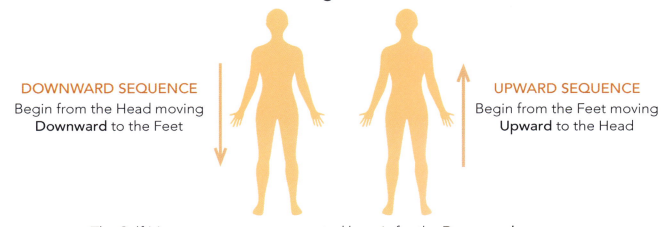

DOWNWARD SEQUENCE
Begin from the Head moving **Downward** to the Feet

UPWARD SEQUENCE
Begin from the Feet moving **Upward** to the Head

The Self Massage sequence presented here is for the **Downward** sequence.
For the **Upward** sequence, simply start at the end of the chapter and work backwards.

Always remember: **DO NOT HURT YOURSELF!**
If you find that a technique is uncomfortable or painful, skip it and move on to another technique.
Everyone is different and not every technique will be appropriate for everyone.

Points used in head massage

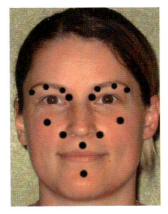 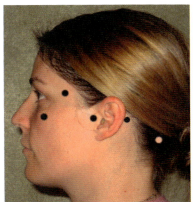 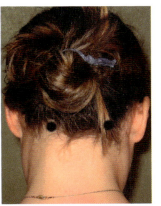 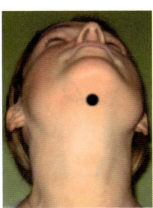

Part I: Self-Massage & Joint Mobilization

SELF MASSAGE – FACE

Face 1

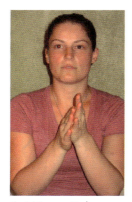
1. Warm Palms

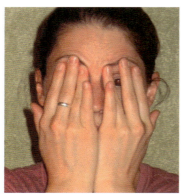
2. Fingertips Below Eyebrows

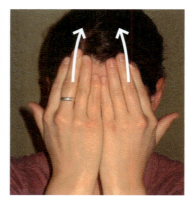
3. To Forehead

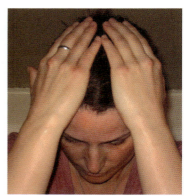
4. Over Scalp

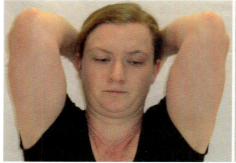
5. Along Back of Neck

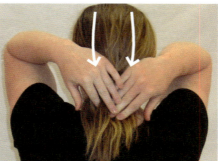

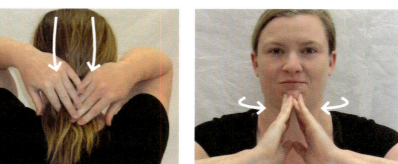
6. Fingers Forward

Face 2

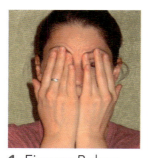
1. Fingers Below Eyebrows

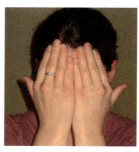
2. Up to Forehead

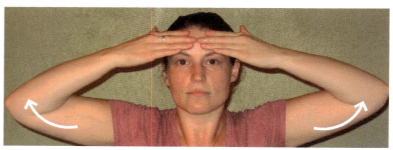
3. Elbows out to Sides, Fingertips Together

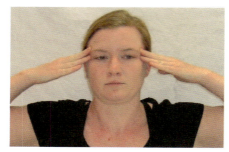
4. Down to Temples

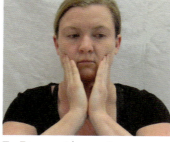
5. Down Along Jaw

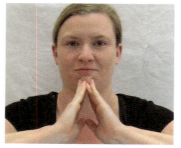
6. To Chin and Out

Traditional Thai Yoga "Reusi Dat Ton"

Face 3

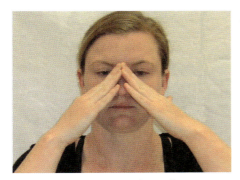
1. Under Eyes & Sides of Nose

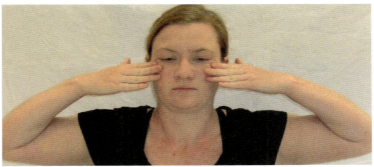
2. Sweep Across Cheeks (Elbows Out to Sides)

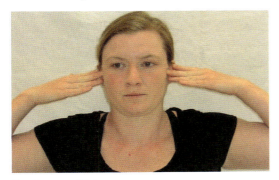
3. Out to Sides

Face 4

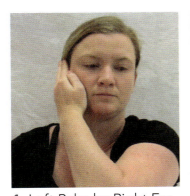
1. Left Palm by Right Ear

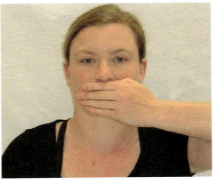
2. Sweep Across Cheeks and Mouth

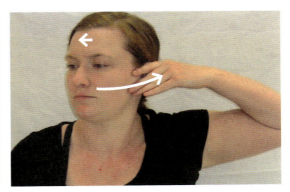
3. To Left Ear

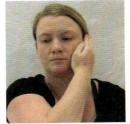 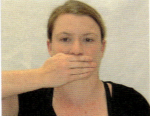 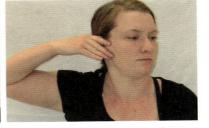

Repeat with Right Hand Sweeping Across Face from Left to Right

Part 1: Self-Massage & Joint Mobilization

Face 5

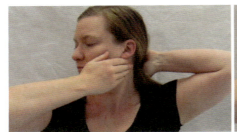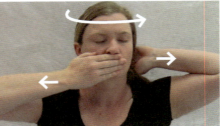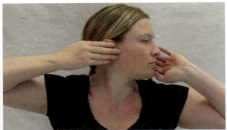

Right Hand Brushes from Left to Right as Head Twists to Left

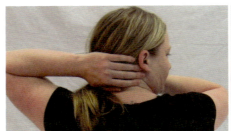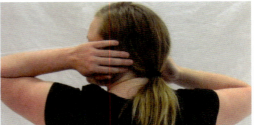

Simultaneously Left Hand Brushes Back of Head From Right to Left

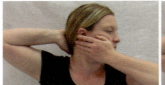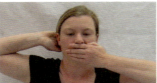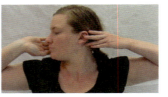

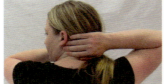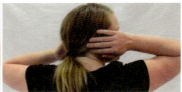

(Repeat on Other Side)

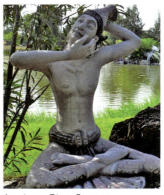

Ancient City, Samut Prakan, Thailand
(Photo Courtesy Heath Reed)

Face 6

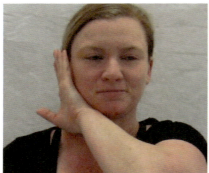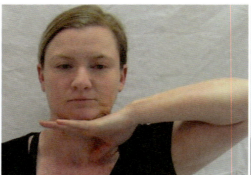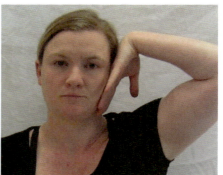

Back of Left Hand Brushes from Right Ear, Under Chin to Left Ear
(Repeat on Other Side)

Traditional Thai Yoga "Reusi Dat Ton"

Ears

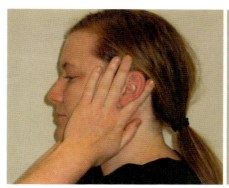 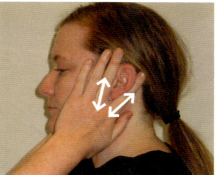

Fingers Massaging Up and Down Ears and Side of Head

Closing The Sense Organs

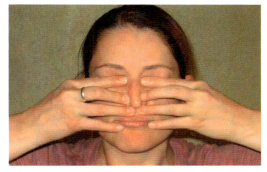 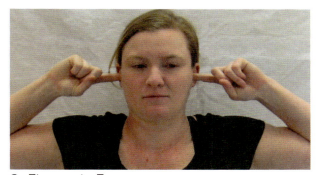

1. Mouth (Little & Ring Fingers)
   Nose (Middle Fingers)
   Eyes (Index Fingers)
   Ears (Thumb Close Tragus)
   Engage Throat & Anal Lock
   Inhale – Close Organs
   Retain Breath – Listen to Heartbeat
   Exhale – Release

2. Fingers in Ears
   Listen to Breathing

Neck 1

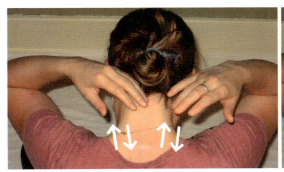 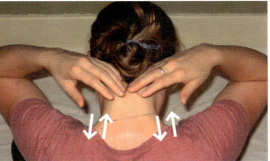

Drop Chin and "Beat" the Neck (Tapotement)

Part 1: Self-Massage & Joint Mobilization

Neck 2

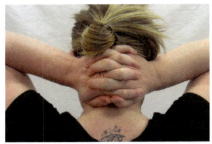
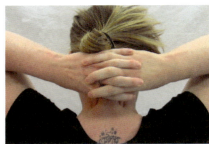
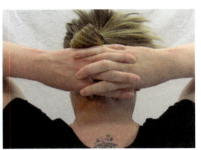

1. Fingers Interlocked Palm Heels Press Side and Back of Neck

2. Thumbs Press Side and Back of Neck

Neck 3

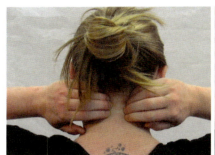
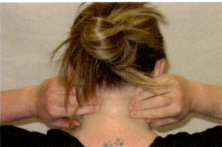
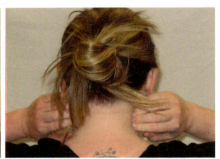

Fingers Glide from Center of Neck Outward

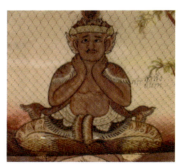

Wat Machimawat Songkhla, Thailand

Neck 4

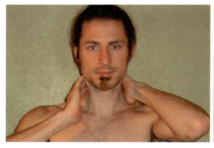
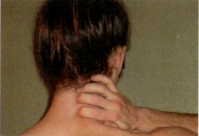
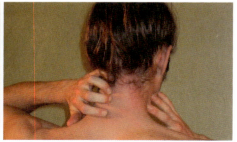

Alternating Fingers Pull from Center Outward

SELF MASSAGE – NECK / SHOULDERS

Neck 5

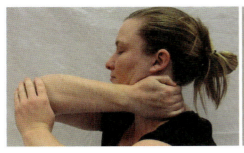 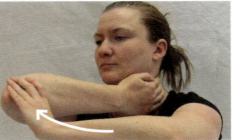

Right Fingers Grab Left Side of Neck,
Left Hand Pushes Right Elbow to Right as Fingers Press into Neck
(Repeat on Other Side)

Pressing the Occiput

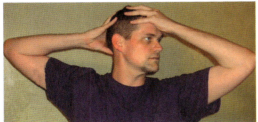 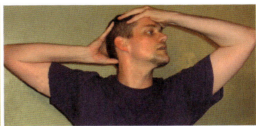 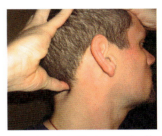

Left Hand to Forehead, Right Thumb to Occiput
Tilt Head Back as Thumb Presses In

Occiput – Below Skull, Outside Perispinal, Inside Trapezius & Sterno Cleido Mastoid

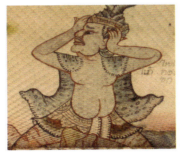

Wat Machimawat
Songkhla, Thailand

Shoulders 1

"For Shoulder Discomfort" Samut Thai Kao (Reusi Dat Ton Manuscript) Circa 1838AD

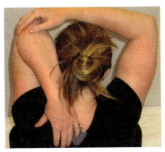 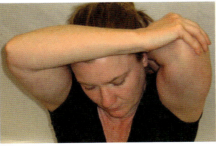 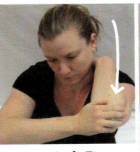 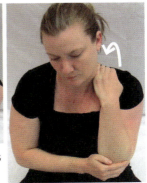

1. Left Hand Grabs Upper Back

2. Right Hand Pushes Left Elbow Down as Left Fingers Glide Up Along Upper Back and onto Shoulder
(Repeat on Other Side)

Part 1: Self-Massage & Joint Mobilization

SELF MASSAGE – SHOULDERS

Shoulders 2

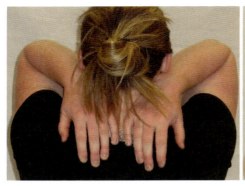 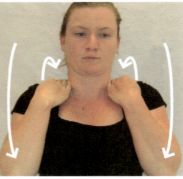

Both Hands Grab Upper Back, Fingers Glide Along Upper Back and onto Shoulders

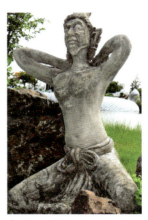

*Ancient City
Samut Prakan, Thailand*

Shoulders 3

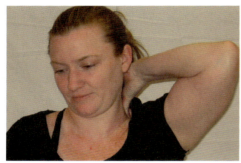 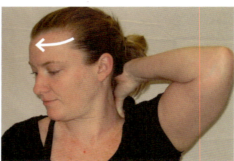

Twist Head to Left. Left Thumb Presses Point Above Collar Bone Below Trapezium Muscle. Twist Head to Right Side.
(Repeat on Other Side)

Shoulders 4

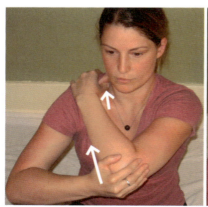 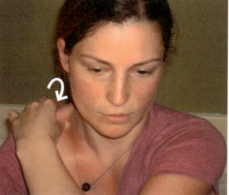

Twist Head to Right. Left Thumb Pushes into Point Above Collar Bone Below Trapezium Muscle with Right Hand Pulling into the Elbow to give more force. Twist Head to Left.
(Repeat on Other Side)

Traditional Thai Yoga "Reusi Dat Ton"

Brush Arm

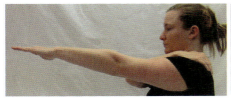 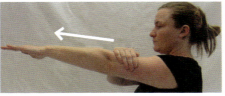 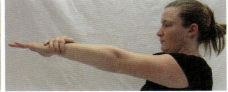

1. Right Palm Brushes Outward Along Top of Left Arm

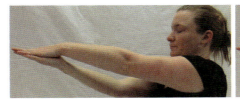 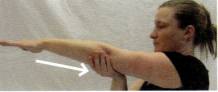 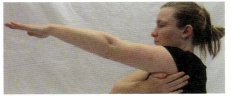

2. Right Palm Brushes Inward Along Bottom of Left Arm

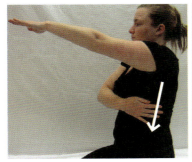 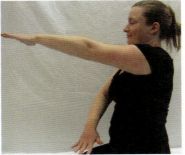

3. Right Palm Brushes Downward Along Left Side of Torso

Beat the Arm

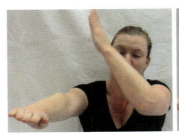 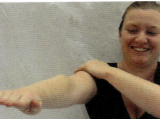 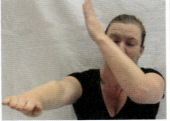 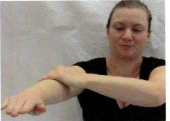

Palm or Fist Vigorously Taps Back & Inside Arm

Arms 1

"For Arm Discomfort" Samut Thai Kao

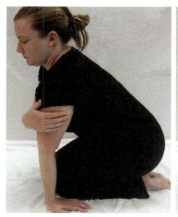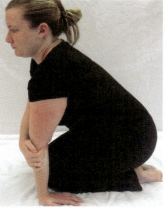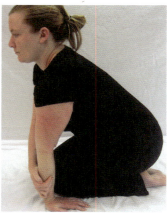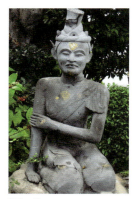

Wat Po, Bangkok, Thailand

1. Left Palm to Floor with Fingers Pointed Back, Right Fingers Massage Up & Down Back of Left Arm

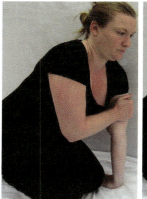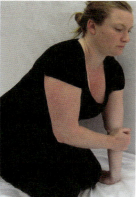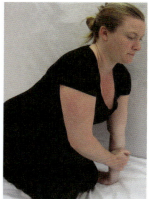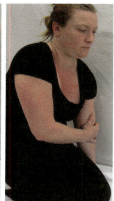

2. Right Thumb or Palm Heel Massage Up & Down Inside of Left Arm

Arms 2

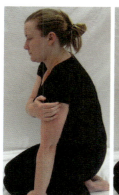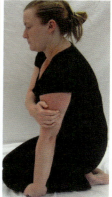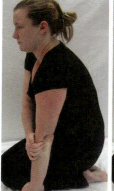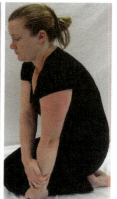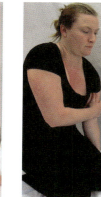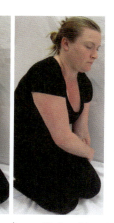

1. Left Hand with Palm Up Pinned Down Under Left Shin, Right Fingers Massage Up & Down Back of Left Arm

2. Right Thumb or Palm Heel Massage Up and Down Inside of Left Arm

Traditional Thai Yoga "Reusi Dat Ton"

SELF MASSAGE – PALMS   23

Palms 1
"For Hand Discomfort" Samut Thai Kao

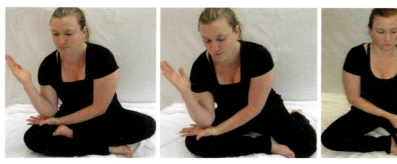

(Seated Cross-Legged or in "Mermaid Pose")
Massage Palm with Elbow, Forearm, and/or Thumb

Palms 2

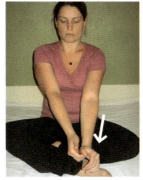 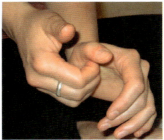

Fingers Curled with Tips to Point
in Palm Webbing, Lever Push Arm

Palms 3

Thumb Gliding Outward Along Trenches of Palm

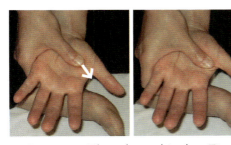 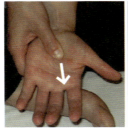 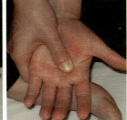

1. Between Thumb and Index Finger   **2.** Between Index and Middle Finger

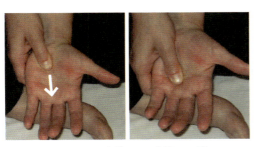 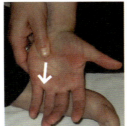 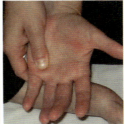

3. Between Middle and Ring Finger   **4.** Between Ring and Little Finger

Part 1: Self-Massage & Joint Mobilization

Fingers

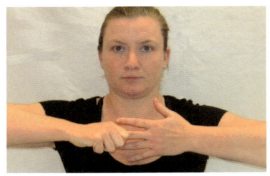 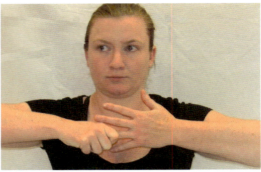

Gently Pull (Mobilize) Fingers
(Repeat Arm, Palm, Hand, and Fingers on Other Side)

Pectorals

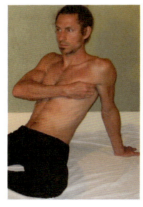 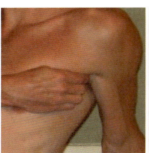 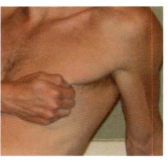 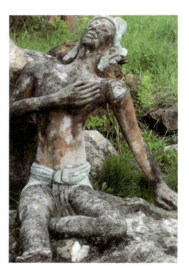

Hand Reaches Across Chest to Massage
Along Outside Edge of Pectorals

Ancient City "Muang Boran," Samut Prakan, Thailand

Belly & Back

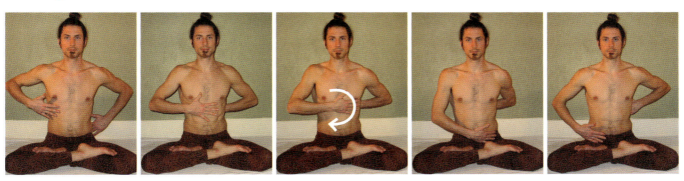

Right Palm Rubs Across Upper Abdomen from Right to Left,
Downward, Then Across Lower Abdomen Left to Right

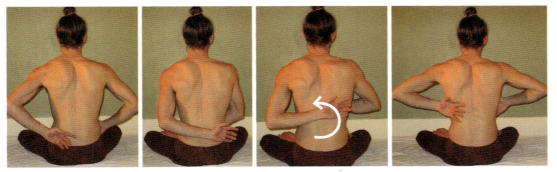

Simultaneously, Back of Left Hand Rubs Across Low Back from Left to Right,
Upward, then Across Mid Back Right to Left

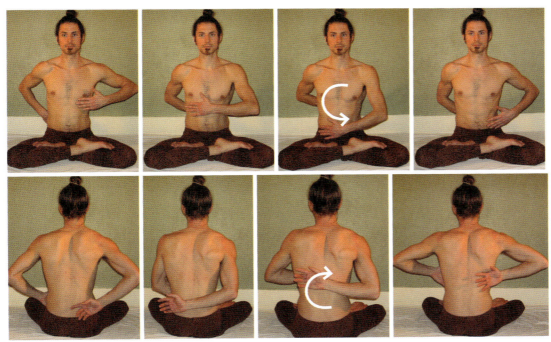

Repeat with Hand Positions Reversed
(Continuing the Cycle)

Back

Knuckles

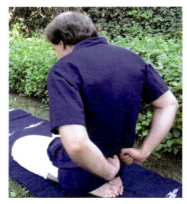
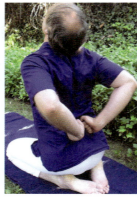
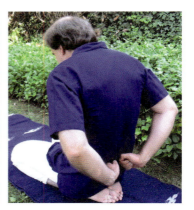

1. Inhale - Slouch   **2.** Exhale - Push In, Look Up   **3.** Inhale - Slouch

Thumbs

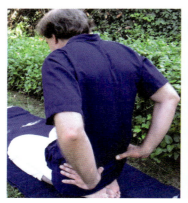
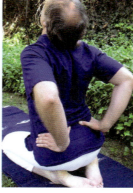
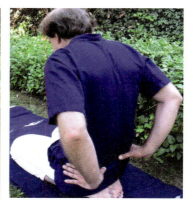

1. Inhale - Slouch   **2.** Exhale - Push In, Look Up   **3.** Inhale - Slouch

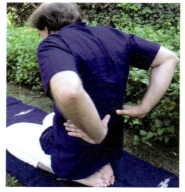
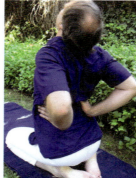
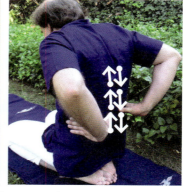

Thumbs Move Up and Down Along Back

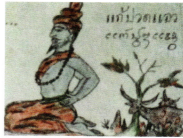

"For Hip and Lower Back Pain"
From a rare "Reusi Dat Ton"
text hand copied by Reusi
Prasanga Samavajra

Traditional Thai Yoga "Reusi Dat Ton"

SELF MASSAGE — TORSO & BACK / LEGS

Beat the Back

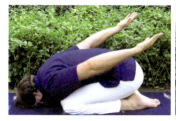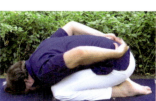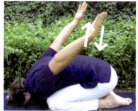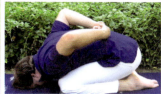

Bend Forward and do Tapotement to Back

Beat the Butt

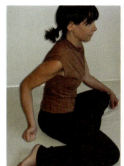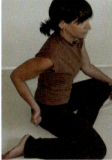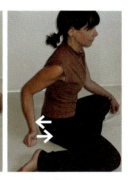

In Mermaid Pose do Tapotement to the Gluteus

Brushing the Legs (Sides)

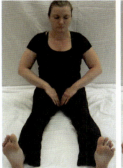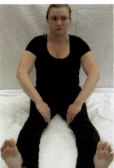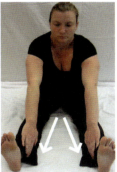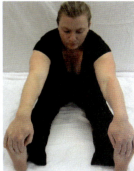

Palms Brush Legs from Inner Thighs Downward to Soles of Feet then

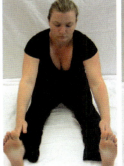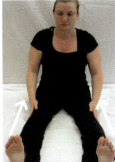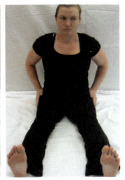

Upward Along Outside of Legs to Hips (Reverse the Pattern)

Part 1: Self-Massage & Joint Mobilization

Brushing the Legs (Tops)

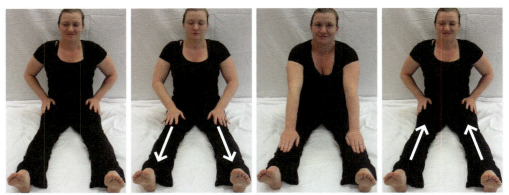

Palms Brush from Top of Thighs Downward to Feet and Back Up

Upper Leg (Inner)

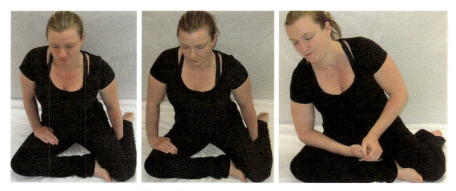

Palm, Forearm, and/or Elbow Pressing Up and Down Inner Thigh

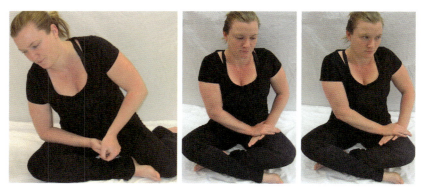

In Mermaid or Cross-Legged

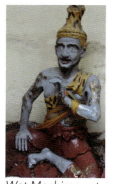

*Wat Machimawat
Songkhla, Thailand*

Traditional Thai Yoga "Reusi Dat Ton"

Upper Leg (Outer)

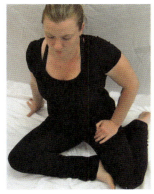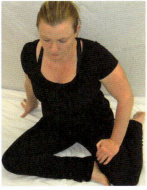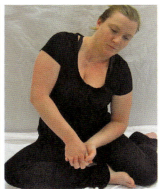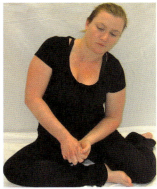

Palm, Forearm, and/or Elbow Pressing Up and Down Outer Thigh

Upper Leg (Back)

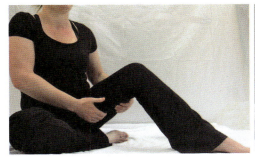

Alternate Finger Pull ("*Unwinding*" in Thai) Up & Down Back of Upper Leg

Upper Leg (Front)

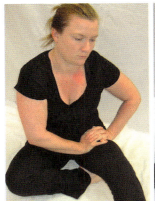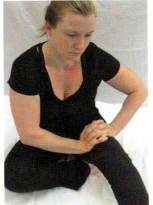

Fingers Interlocked, Palm Heels Pressing Up and Down Front of Upper Leg and Down Outer Thigh

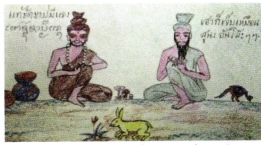

"*For Poor Circulation and Leg Weakness*"
From a rare "*Reusi Dat Ton*" text hand copied by Reusi Prasanga Samavajra

Part 1: Self-Massage & Joint Mobilization

Lower Leg (Back)

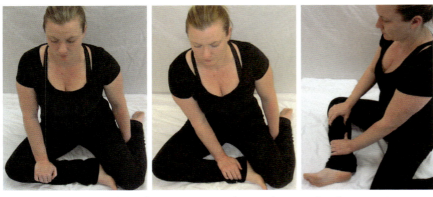

1. Palm Heel or Thumbs Pressing Along the Back of Lower Leg

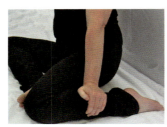 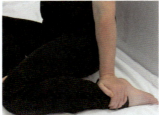

2. In Mermaid Pose, Palm Heel Pressing Along Back of Lower Leg

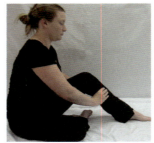 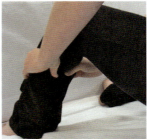

3. With Knee Up, Thumbs Pressing Along Back of Lower Leg

Lower Leg (Front)

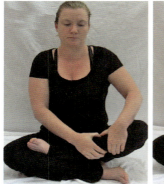 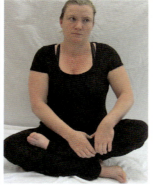

1. Fingers Pressing Along Front of Lower Leg

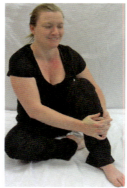 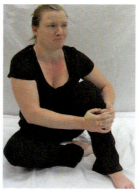

2. Fingers Interlocked, Palm Heels Pressing Along Lower Leg

Feet 1

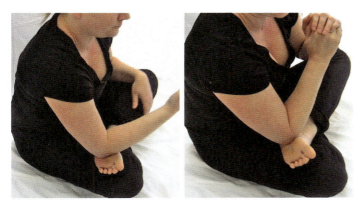

Elbow and Forearm Pressing Sole of Foot

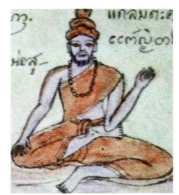

"For Cramps"
From a rare "Reusi Dat Ton" text hand copied by Reusi Prasanga Samavajra

Feet 2

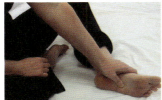 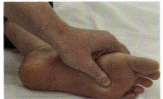

1. Thumb to Sole of Foot

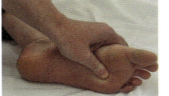 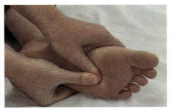

2. Two Thumbs to Sole of Foot

Feet 3

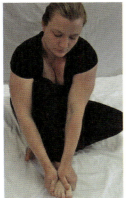 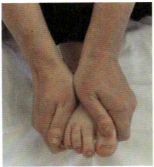 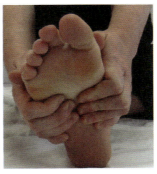

Fingers to Sole of Foot as Palm Heels or Thumbs Press Instep

Part I: Self-Massage & Joint Mobilization

Toes 1

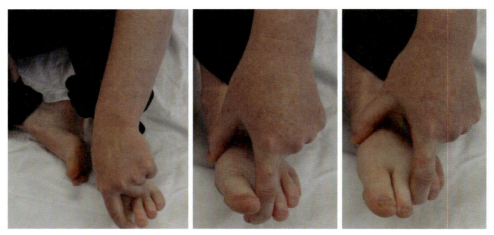

Gently Mobilize (Pull or Bend) Toes One by One

Toes 2

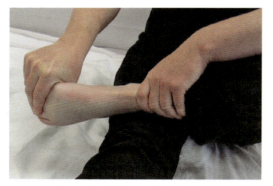

Bend All Toes Together

Repeat Legs, Feet, and Toes on Other Side,
So that Both Sides of the Body Have Been Done

Sen Lines of Northern Thai "Lanna" Massage

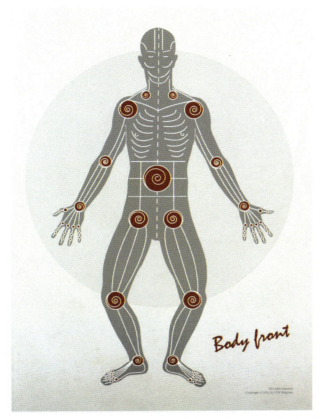

Body front

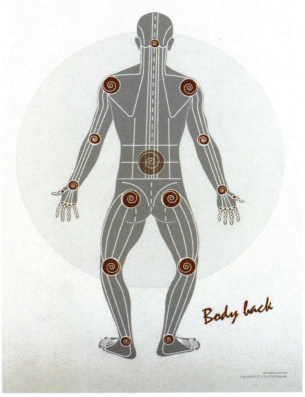

Body back

(Charts Courtesy of Danko Lara Radic, Institute of Thai Massage, Belgrade)

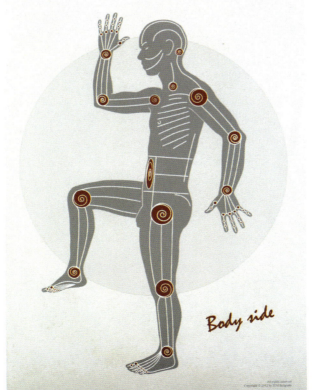

Body side

Joint Mobilization
"Shaking the Joints"

"Reusi Dat Ton exercises help to clear the wind pathways of obstructions and balance the breathwinds. They correct any sort of imbalance in the structure, open the joints, make the tissues more malleable, and open the channels, helping to calm and manage the wind."

– Reusi Tevijjo

Clears stagnant Wind from the Joints, Improves Range of Motion and Circulation, Increases Lubrication (Synovial Fluid) in the Joints.

EACH MOVEMENT A MINIMUM OF 21 TIMES.
Over time and with practice, one can gradually build up to more 50, 108… for Therapeutic Purposes. These sequences can be done either sitting or standing.

UPPER BODY
Begin from **Center**
Moving **Outward**
Shoulders out to Fingers

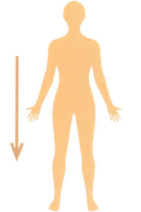

DOWNWARD SEQUENCE
Begin with Upper Body moving **Downward** to Hips continuing down Legs to Toes

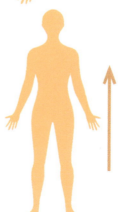

UPWARD SEQUENCE
Begin with Toes moving **Upward** to Hips, continuing Up to Upper Body

Always remember: **DO NOT HURT YOURSELF!**
If you find that a technique is uncomfortable or painful, skip it and move on to another technique. Everyone is different and not every technique will be appropriate for everyone.

Traditional Thai Yoga "Reusi Dat Ton"

Seated Joint Mobilization

The Seated Joint Mobilization sequence presented here is for the **Upward** sequence. For the **Downward** sequence, simply start at the end of this section and work backwards.

Toes

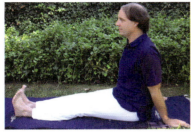 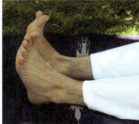 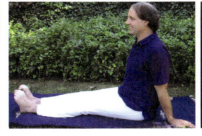 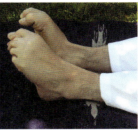

1. Spread Toes Upward   **2.** Curl Toes Downward

Ankles

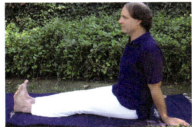 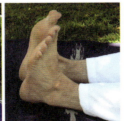 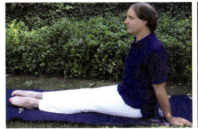 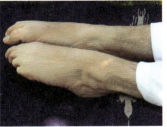

1. Feet Upward   **2.** Feet Downward

Knees

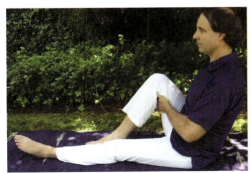 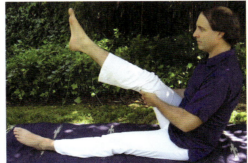

1. Bend Leg – Full Flexion   **2.** Straighten Leg – Full Extension

(Repeat on Other Leg)

Part I: Self-Massage & Joint Mobilization

Hips

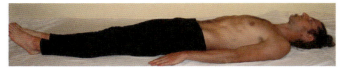

1. Reclining on Back

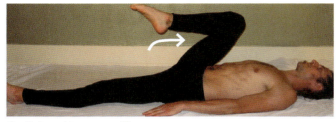

2. Bring Knee to Chest

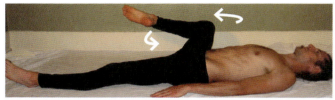

3. Circle Knee Out to Side then Straighten Leg Back to Starting Position

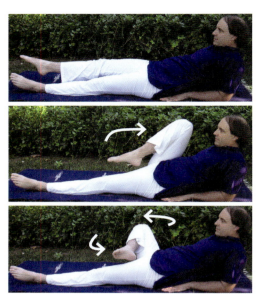

(May also be done Seated or Reclining on Elbows, with Leg Bent as shown here or with Leg Straight)

(Circle Same Leg Opposite Direction, Then Repeat on Other Leg)

Torso

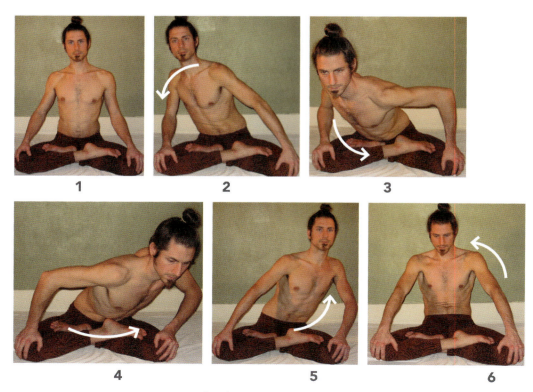

Circle Torso (Both Directions)

Traditional Thai Yoga "Reusi Dat Ton"

Ribs

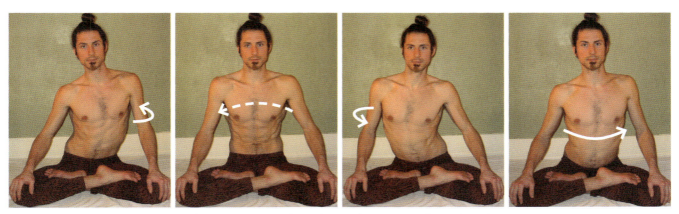

Seated Cross Legged, Isolate Ribcage and Circle Ribcage
(As if Swirling Wine Around the Inside of a Wineglass)
(Both Directions)

Trunk Twisting

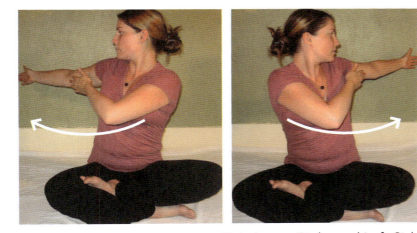
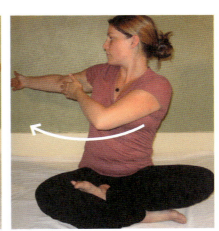

Twisting to Right and Left Sides

JOINT MOBILIZATION

Shoulders 1

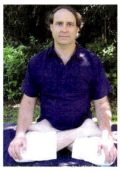
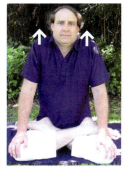
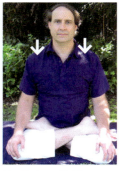
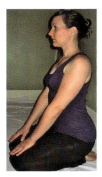

1. Relax **2.** Shoulders Up **3.** Relax & Drop

These Exercises may also be done Kneeling

Shoulders 2

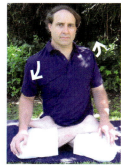
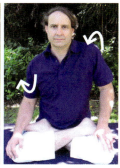
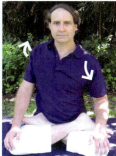
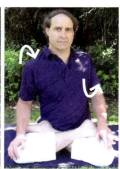

Circling Each Shoulder Opposite the Other ("Kayak Like")
(Then Reverse, Circling in Opposite Directions)

Shoulders 3

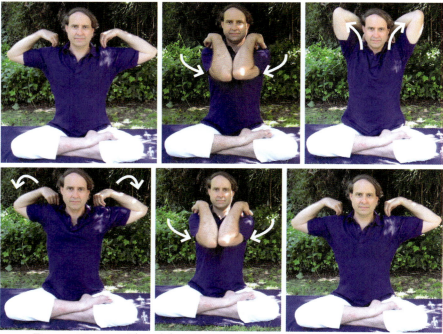

Finger Tips to Shoulder Joints, Circle Elbows Out at Sides
(Circle Opposite Direction)

Traditional Thai Yoga "Reusi Dat Ton"

Elbows

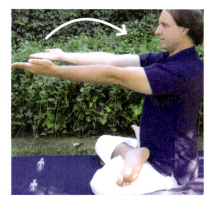 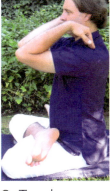 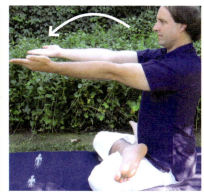

1. Arms Straight (Full Extension)
2. Touch Shoulders (Full Flexion)
3. Straighten Arms (Full Extension)

Wrists

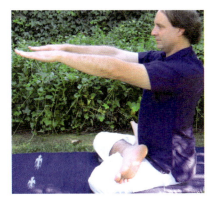 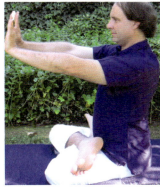 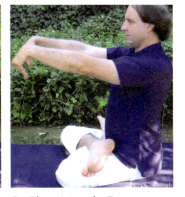

1. Extend Hands
2. Flap Hands Up
3. Flap Hands Down

Fingers

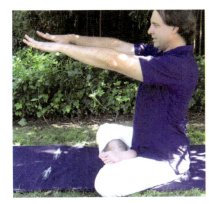 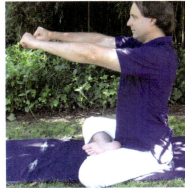 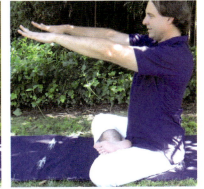

1. Extend Fingers
2. Fingertips to Palms
3. Extend Fingers

(One may then again "Pull or Mobilize the Fingers" as shown after Hand Massage)

Part I: Self-Massage & Joint Mobilization

Neck

"For Bad Wind in the Neck"   Samut Thai Kao (Reusi Dat Ton Manuscript) Circa 1838AD

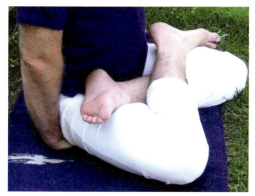

Sit on Back of Hands, Palms Down
(Sit Tall and Straight)

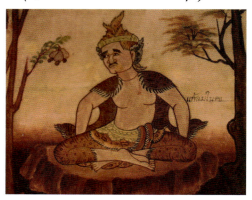

Wat Machimawat, Songkhla, Thailand

Neck 1

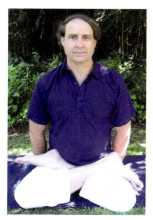 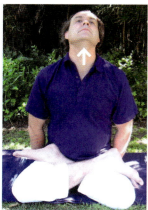 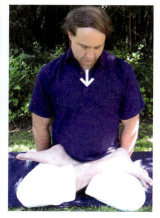

1. Sit on Hands   **2.** Chin Up   **3.** Chin Down

Neck 2

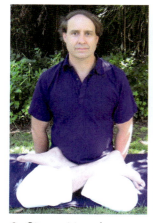 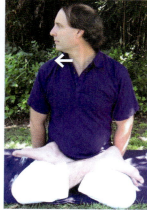 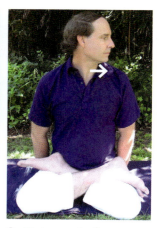

1. Sit on Hands   **2.** Twist to Right   **3.** Twist to Left

Traditional Thai Yoga "Reusi Dat Ton"

Neck 3

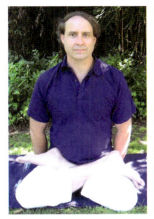 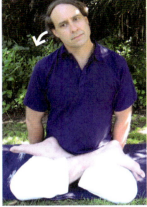 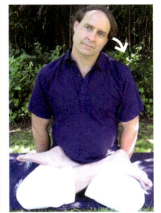

1. Sit on Hands **2.** Head to Right **3.** Head to Left

Neck 4

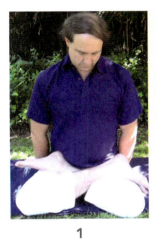 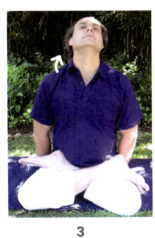 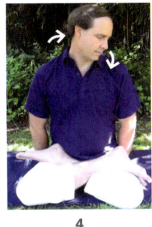

1 2 3 4

Slowly Circle Head (Both Directions)

Jaw

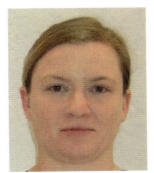 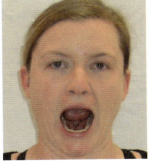

Open and Close Jaw

Eyes

Careful to Only Move the Eyes, the Head Remains Stationary
(Repeat Eye Movements 21X for Each Exercise)

1

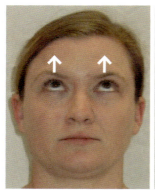 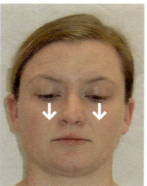

Look Up and Down

2

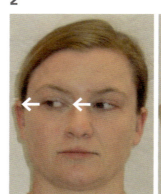 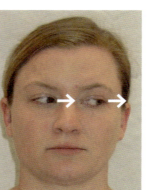

Look Right and Left

3

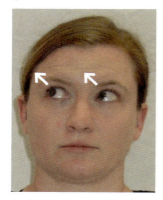 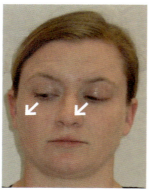 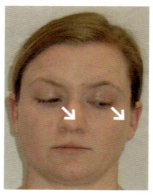 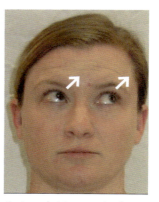

1. Look Upper Right **2.** Look Lower Right **3.** Look Lower Left **4.** Look Upper Left

Eyes Look at the Four Corners of an Invisible Square
(Repeat in Opposite Direction)

Standing Joint Mobilization

The Standing Joint Mobilization presented here is for the **Downward** sequence.
For the **Upward** sequence, simply start at the end of this section and work backwards.

Neck

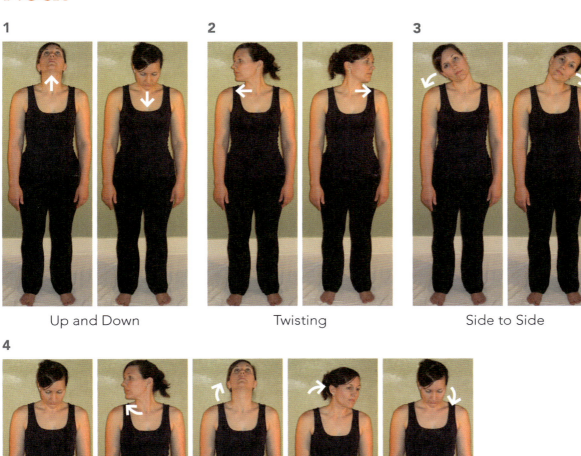

1. Up and Down
2. Twisting
3. Side to Side
4. Circle (Both Directions)

Part 1: Self-Massage & Joint Mobilization

Jaw

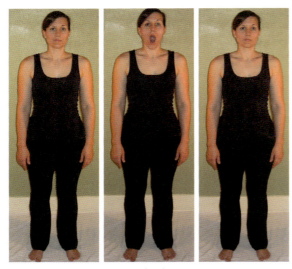

Open and Close Jaw

Eyes

Careful to Only Move the Eyes, the Head Remains Stationary
(Repeat Eye Movements 21X for Each Exercise)

1

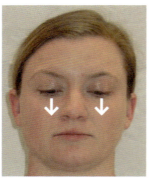

Look Up and Down

2

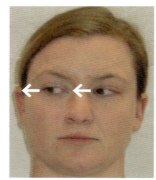

Look Right and Left

3

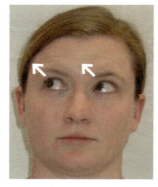 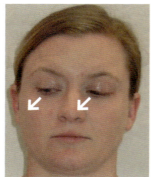 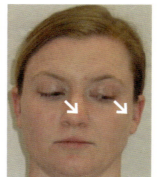 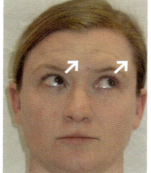

1. Look Upper Right **2.** Look Lower Right **3.** Look Lower Left **4.** Look Upper Left

Eyes Look at the Four Corners of an Invisible Square
(Repeat in Opposite Direction)

Traditional Thai Yoga "Reusi Dat Ton"

Shoulder Shrugs

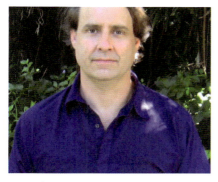
1. Relax

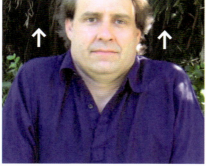
2. Tense, Shoulders Up

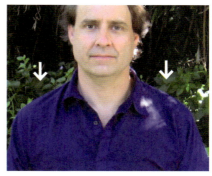
3. Relax & Drop

Shoulder Rolls

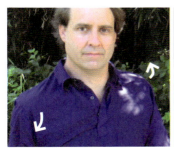 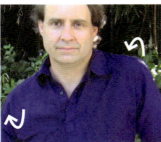 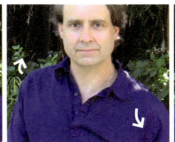 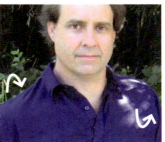

Circling Each Shoulder Opposite the Other ("Kayak Like")
(Then Reverse, Circling in Opposite Directions)

Arm Circles

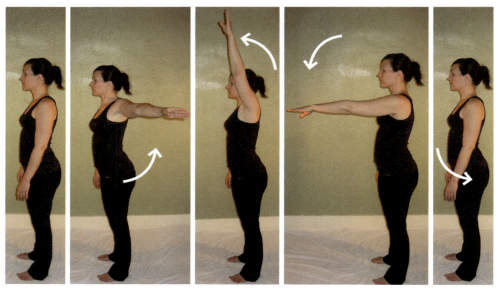

Circle One Arm 21 X Each Way (Then Circle Other Arm 21 X Each Way)

Elbows

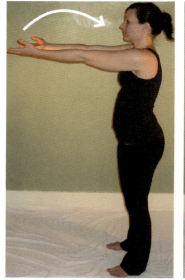
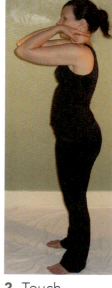
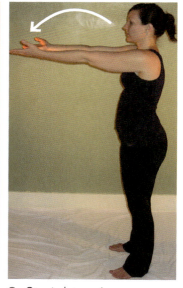

1. Arms Straight **2.** Touch Shoulders **3.** Straighten Arms

Wrists

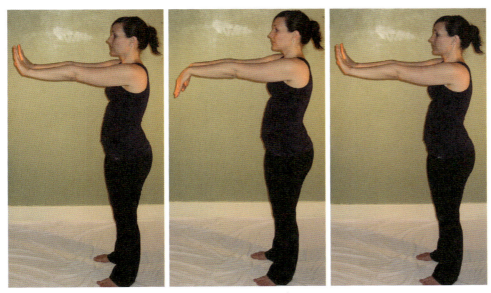

Wrists Flap Up and Down

Fingers

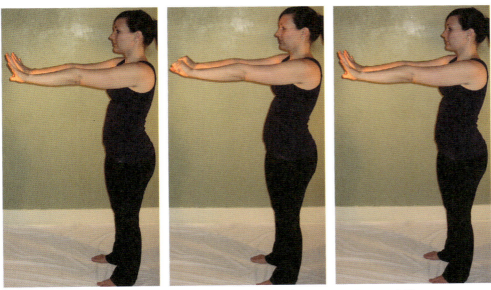

1. Extend Fingers   **2.** Fingertips to Palms   **3.** Extend Fingers

(One may then again "Pull or Mobilize the Fingers" as shown after Hand Massage)

Trunk Twisting

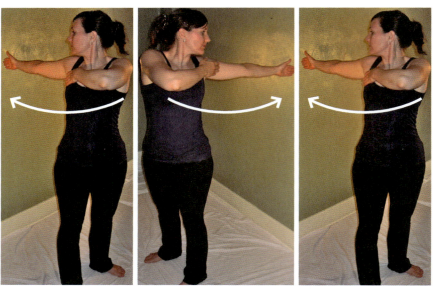
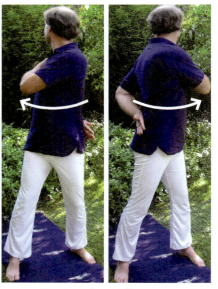

Twisting to Right and Left Sides

(In Confined Spaces Arms May be Bent)

Ribs

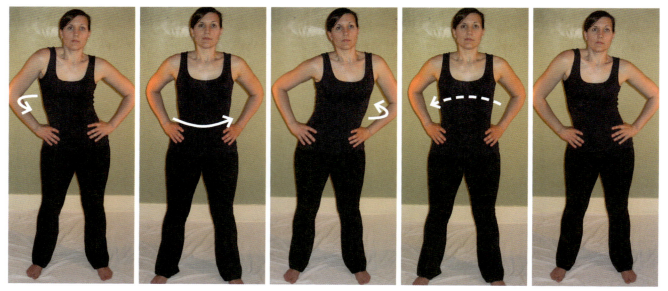

Isolate Ribcage and Circle Ribcage (As if Swirling Wine Around the Inside of a Wineglass)
(Circle Both Directions)

Hips

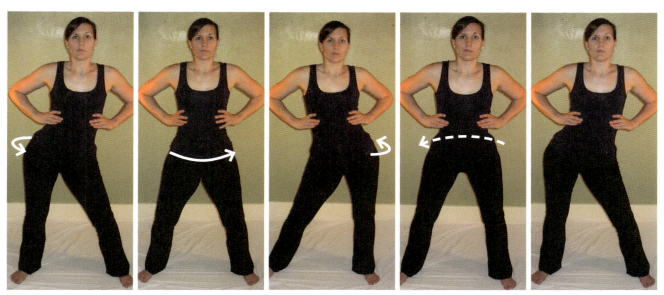

Isolate Hips and Circle

(Both Directions)

Torso

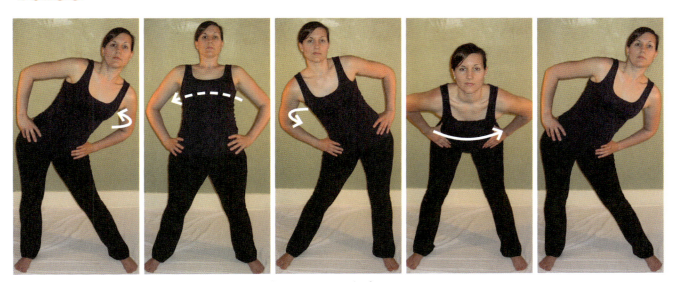

Circle Entire Body from Hips

(Circle Both Directions)

Part 1: Self-Massage & Joint Mobilization

Hips

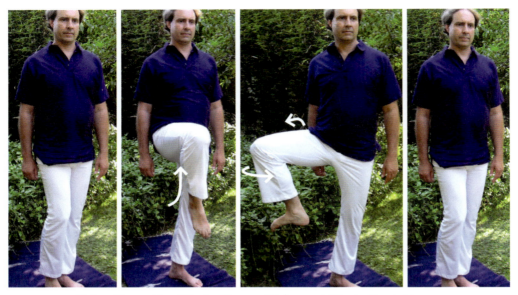

Raise Knee Up, Circle Out to Side and Circle Back Down
(Circle Other Direction, Then Circle Other Leg Both Ways)

Knees

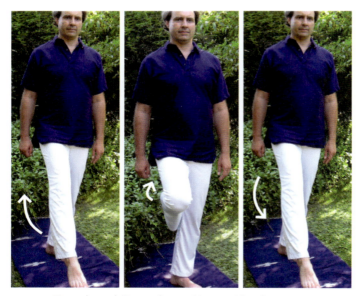

Bend and Straighten Knee, Heel to Hip
(Full Extension and Flexion)

Ankles

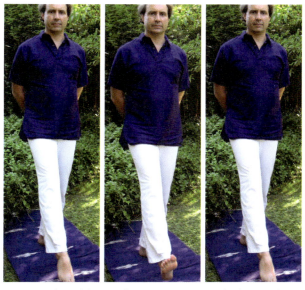
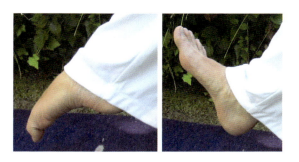

Bend Ankle (Full Extension and Flexion)

Toes

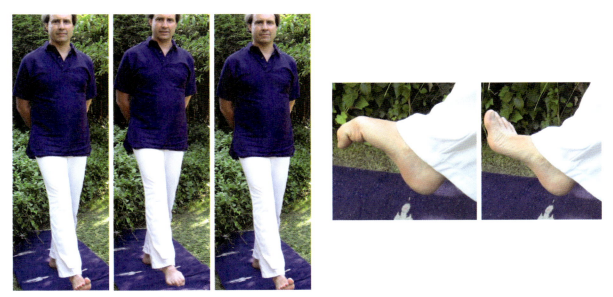

Bend Toes

(One may then again "Bend or Mobilize the Toes" as shown after Foot Massage)

Part I: Self-Massage & Joint Mobilization

References

English Language

Baker, Ian A. and Thomas Laird. (2000). "The Dali Lama's Secret Temple: Tantric Wall Paintings from Tibet." Thames & Hudson Ltd., London, UK.

Buhnemann, Gudrun. (2007). "Eighty-Four Asanas in Yoga: A Survey of Traditions." (Contains the *Jogapradipika of Jayatarama*). D. K. Printworld, New Delhi, India.

Chokevivat, Vichai and Chuthaputti, Anchalee. (2005). "The Role of Thai Traditional Medicine in Health Promotion." Thai Ministry of Public Health, Nonthaburi, Thailand.

Chuthaputti, Anchalee. (2007). "National Traditional System of Medicine Recognized by the Thai Government." Thai Ministry of Public Health, Nonthaburi, Thailand.

Covington, Laura. (2010). "Interview with a Reusi." (Interview with Reusi Tevijjo). Bodhi Tree Learning Center. Richmond, USA.

Evans-Wentz, W. Y. (2006). "Tibetan Yoga and Secret Doctrines." Pilgrims Publishing, Varanasi, India.

Gharote, M. L. (Editor). (2013). "Encyclopaedia of Traditional Asanas." The Lonavala Yoga Institute. Lonavala, India.

Ginsburg, Henry. (2000). "Thai Art and Culture: Historic Manuscripts from Western Collections." University of Hawaii, Honolulu, USA.

Griswold, A.B. (1965). "The Rishis of Wat Po." *In Felicitation Volumes of Southeast Asian Studies Presented to His Highness Prince Dhaninivat Kromamun Bidyalabh Brindhyakorn*. The Siam Society, Bangkok, Thailand.

H.H. Prince Dhani Nivat, "The Inscriptions of Wat Phra Jetubon," *Journal of the Siam Society.* Vol. 26, Pt. 2. The Siam Society, Bangkok, Thailand.

Hofbauer, Rudolf. "A Medical Retrospect of Thailand." In Journal of the Thailand Research Society, 34: 183-200. Thailand Research Society, Bangkok, Thailand.

Linrothe, Rob, (Editor). (2006). "Holy Madness: Portraits of Tantric Siddhas." Rubin Museum of Art and Serindia Publications. New York and Chicago, USA.

Mallinson, James. (2012). "Yoga and Yogis." Namarupa, Categories of Indian Thought, Issue 15, Volume 3, March 2012.

Miao, Yuan. (2002). "Dancing on Rooftops with Dragons: The Yoga of Joy." The Philosophical Research Society, Los Angeles, USA.

Matics, Kathleen Isabelle. (1978). *An Historical Analysis of the Fine Arts at Wat Phra Chetuphon: A Repository of Ratanakosin Artistic Heritage*, PhD Dissertation, New York University, New York, USA.

Matics, K.I. (1977). "Medical Arts at Wat Pha Chetuphon: Various Rishi Statues." In *Journal of the Siam Society*, 65:2: 2: 145-152. The Siam Society, Bangkok, Thailand.

Norbu, Chogyal Namkhai. (2008). "Yantra Yoga: The Tibetan Yoga of Movement." Snow Lion Publications, Ithaca, USA.

Reusi Tevijo Yogi. Personal Communication. Bangkok and Chiang Mai, Thailand.

Salguero, C. Pierce, (2007). "Traditional Thai Medicine: Buddhism, Animism and Ayurveda." Hohm Press, Prescott, USA.

Saraswati, Swami Satyananda. (2006). "Asana, Pranayama, Mudra, Bandha." Bihar School of Yoga, Yoga Publications Trust, Munger, India.

Schoeppl, Adolf. (1981). *Textbook of Thai Traditional Manipulative Medicine*, MPH Thesis, Mahidol University, Bangkok, Thailand.

Sheposh, Joel. (2006). *Reusi Dat Ton: Thai Style Exercises*, Tao Mt. Chatlottesville, USA.

Subcharoen, Pennapa and Deewised Kunchana, (Editors). (1995). "The Hermits Art of Contorting: Thai Traditional Medicine." The National Institute of Thai Traditional Medicine, Nontaburi, Thailand.

The Thai Massage School of Chiang Mai. (2006). *Yogi Exercise "Lue Sri Dadton" Student Handbook*. Massage School of Chiang Mai, Chiang Mai, Thailand.

Tulku, Tarthang. (1978). "Kum Nye Relaxation: Parts 1and 2." Dharma Publishing, Berkeley, USA.

Tulku, Tarthang. (2003). "Tibetan Relaxation: Kum Nye Massage and Movement." Duncan Baird Publications, London, UK.

Venerable Dhammasaro Bhikkhu. "Textbook of Basic Physical Training- Hermit Style (Rishi)." Wat Po. Bangkok, Thailand.

Wat Po Thai Traditional Medical School, *Ruesi Dat Ton; Student Handbook*. Wat Po. Bangkok, Thailand.

White, David Gordon. (1996). "The Alchemical Body: Siddha Traditions in Medieval India." University of Chicago Press, Chicago, USA

REFERENCES

Thai Language

Ajan Pisit Benjamongkonware. (2007). "Twenty One Self Stretching Exercises *(21 Ta Dat Ton)*." Village Doctor Press, Bangkok, Thailand.

Ajan Pisit Benjamongkonware. Personal Communication. Pisit's Massage School, Bangkok, Thailand,

Ajan Kong Kaew Veera Prajak (Professor of Ancient Languages). Personal Communication. The Ancient Manuscript and Inscription Department, National Library, Bangkok, Thailand.

Chaya, Ooh E. (2006). "Thai Massage, Reusi Dat Ton: Therapy for Illness and Relaxation, *(Nuat Thai, Reusi Dat Ton: Bam Bat Rok Pai Klie Klieat)*." Pi Rim Press, Bangkok, Thailand.

Karen Reusi. Personal Communication via Dr. Robert Steinmetz of Wildlife Fund Thailand. Thung Yai National Park in Kanchanaburi Province, Thailand,

Mr. Kayat, (Editor). (1995). "Eighty Poses of Reusi Dat Ton, Wat Po *(80 Ta Bat Reusi Dat Ton, Wat Po)*." Pee Wa Tin Press, Bangkok, Thailand.

Mulaniti Health Center. (1994). "41 Poses, The Art of Self Massage for Health, *(41 Ta, Sinlaba Gan Nuat Don Eng Pua Sukapap)*." Mulaniti Health Center, Bangkok, Thailand.

Patanagit, Arun Rawee. (1994). "Body Exercise, Thai Style: Reusi Dat Ton, *(Gan Brehan Rang Gie Bap Thai: Chut Reusi Dat Ton)*." Petchkarat Press. Bangkok, Thailand.

Saw Pai Noie. (2001). *"Lang Neua Chop Lang Ya."* Sai Ton Press, Bangkok, Thailand.

Sela Noie, Laeiat. (2000). "Amazing Thai Heritage: Reusi Dat Ton." Dok Ya Press, Bangkok, Thailand.

Subcharoen, Pennapa (Editor). (2004). "Handbook of Thai Style Exercise: 15 Basic Reusi Dat Ton Poses, *(Ku Mu Gie Brehan Bap Thai Reusi Dat Ton 15 Ta)*." Thai Traditional Medicine Development Foundation, Bangkok, Thailand.

Subcharoen, Pennapa (Editor). (2006). "One Hundred Twenty Seven Thai Style Exercises, Reusi Dat Ton *(127 Ta Gie Brehan Bap Thai, Reusi Dat Ton)*." Thai Traditional Medicine Development Foundation, Bangkok, Thailand.

Various authors commissioned by King Rama III. (1838). "The Book of Eighty Rishis Performing Posture Exercises to Cure Various Ailments *(Samut Rup Reusi Dat Ton Kae Rok Tang Tang Baet Sip Rup)*." (Also known as *Samut Thai Kao*) Housed in the National Library Bangkok, Thailand,

Wat Po Thai Traditional Medicine School. (1990). "Reusi Dat Ton Handbook *(Dam Ra Reusi Dat Ton Wat Po)*." (Reproductions from the original Samut Thai Kao). Wat Po Press, Bangkok, Thailand.

Wat Po Thai Traditional Medicine School. (1958). *"The Book Of Medicine (Dam Ra Ya)."* (Contains a Reusi Dat Ton section based on the same verses as the 1838 manuscript, *Samut Thai Kao*, but with completely different illustrations). Wat Po Press, Bangkok, Thailand.

Weerapong Chidnok, Opor Weerapun, Chanchira Wasuntarawat, Parinya Lertsinthai and Ekawee Sripariwuth. (2007). "Effect of Ruesi-Dudton-Stretching-Exercise Training to Anaerobic Fitness in Healthy Sedentary Females." *Naresuan University Journal* 2007; 15 (3) 205-214. Phittsanulok, Thailand.

Printed in Great Britain
by Amazon